LOOK AFTER YOURSELF

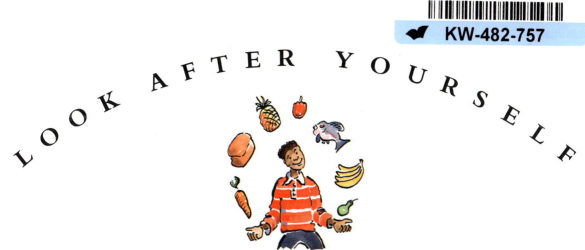

Healthy Food

Anne Qualter & John Quinn

Wayland

Other titles in series

Stay Fit!
Keep Clean!
Stay Safe!

Series editor: Catherine Baxter
Design: Loraine Hayes
Illustration: John Yates/Alan Preston
Photo stylist: Zoë Hargreaves

First published in 1993 by
Wayland (Publishers) Limited,
61 Western Road, Hove,
East Sussex, BN3 1JD, England.
© Copyright 1993 Wayland (Publishers) Ltd.

British Library Cataloguing in Publication Data
Quinn, John
  Healthy Food.—(Look After Yourself Series)
  I.Title II. Qualter, Anne III. Series
  613.2

ISBN 0 7502 0870 8

Typeset by Dorchester Typesetting Group
Limited
Printed and bound in Great Britain by B.P.C.C.
Paulton Books

Photographs by permission of: Chapel Studios 6, 7, 9, 12, 13, 14, 15, 16, 20, 21, 25, 27; Sally and Richard Greenhill 22; Tony Stone 5 (Peter Correz); WPL 23 (top/bottom), 24; Zefa 11 (top, J Tobias/bottom), 18 (Hackenberg), 26 (Parker).

Contents

Growing

Your body is made up of lots of different parts. You have skin, muscles and bones. Can you think of any other parts?

All the time that you are a child, your body is growing. So you need to make more of the different body parts – more skin, more muscle, more bone.

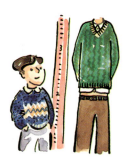

Children don't all grow at the same speed, so don't worry if you're not as tall as your best friend. ▶

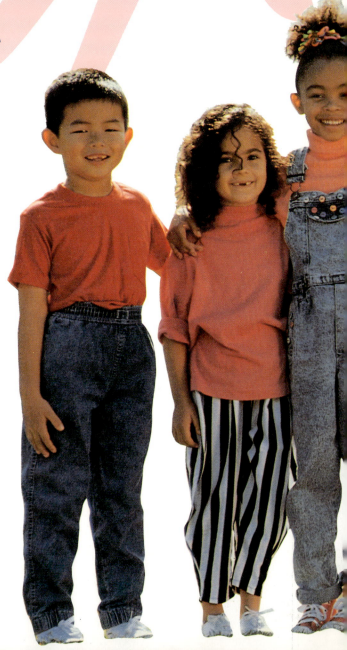

Measure your hand against the toddler's hand on page 4. Is it bigger? Now measure your hand against the grown-up's hand on this page. Is it smaller?

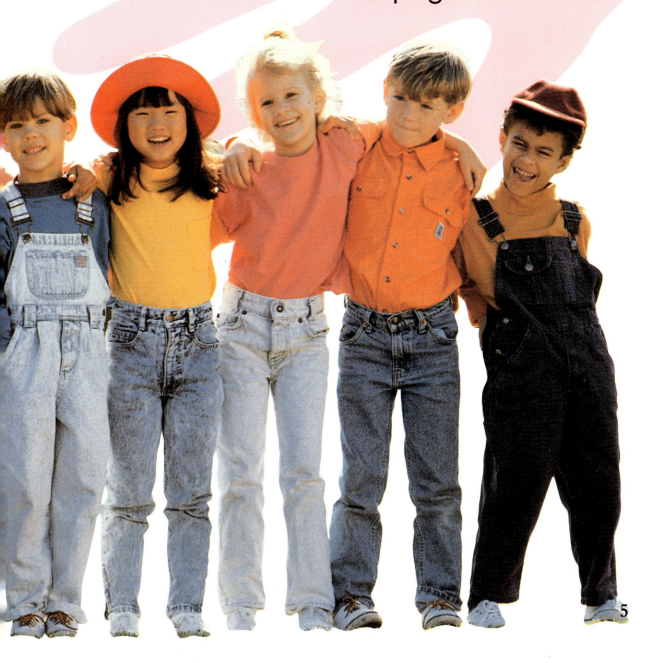

Body cells

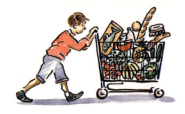

Have you ever built a house out of Lego? You need different bits for the walls, roof, doors and windows. ▼

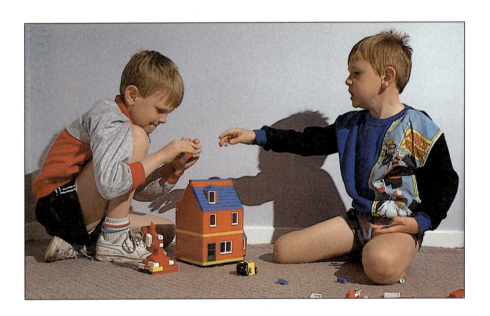

Your body is built of tiny cells. Cells are a bit like the building blocks of your body. You need different cells to make up the different parts of your body – skin cells, muscle cells, bone cells.

WOW!
The Pygmy shrew has to eat three-quarters of its whole body weight each day just to keep going. Imagine how much food we would need if we had to eat three-quarters of our body weight.

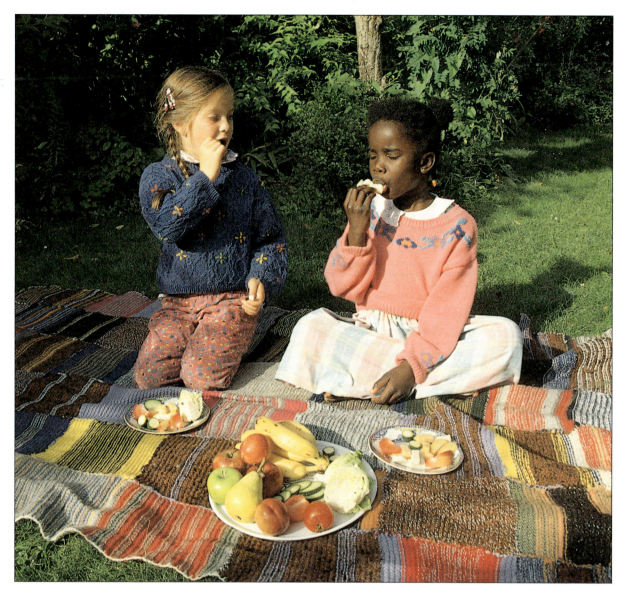

▲ Your body turns the different kinds of food you eat into different cells. Your body breaks up the food into bits, and builds them into parts that you need.

You are always wearing some parts out, so they need to be replaced.

A balanced diet

Your body needs different kinds of food to build into different body parts. You also need food to give you energy to do things.

You need energy to walk to school and energy to climb the stairs. In fact, you even need energy to read this book!

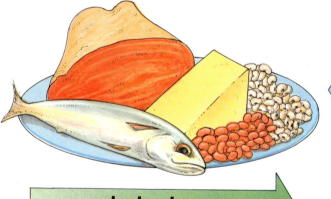

proteins
joint of meat, cheese, fish, black-eye beans, kidney beans

carbohydrates
bread, rice, pasta, potatoes

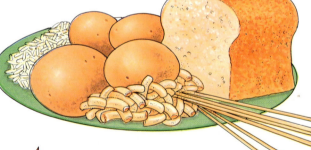

fats
butter, cream, cheese, biscuits, cake

Here are the three main kinds of food you need. ▲

You need to eat just enough food to give you energy, and just enough to make you grow and repair your worn-out parts. We call this having a balanced diet.

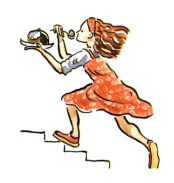

Get a grown-up to cut out several round plate shapes from a large piece of paper. Draw some of your favourite meals on the paper plates. Which food types do your meals contain? ▼

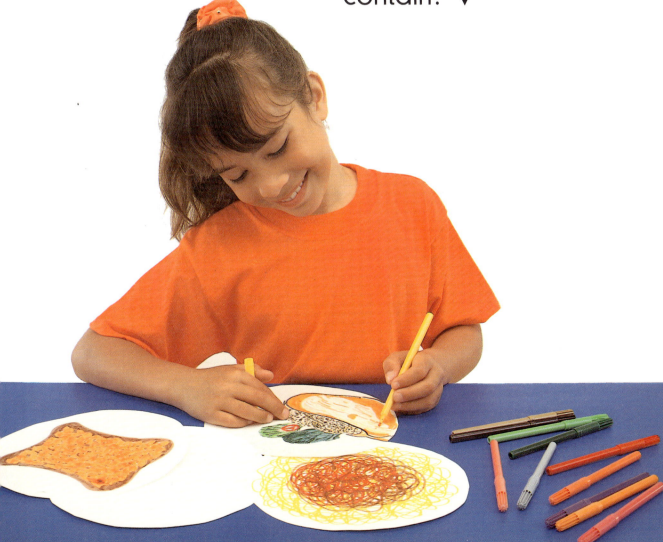

Energy

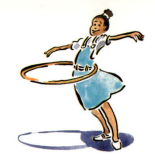

Different things you do use different amounts of energy. This chart shows you which kinds of activities need the most energy. ▼

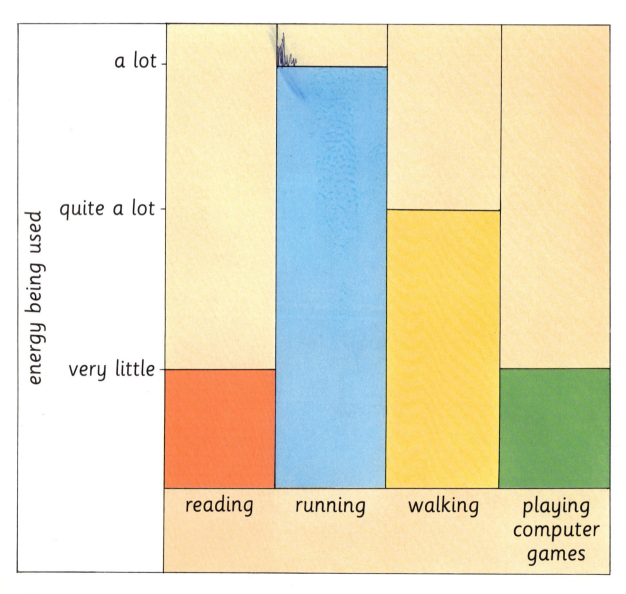

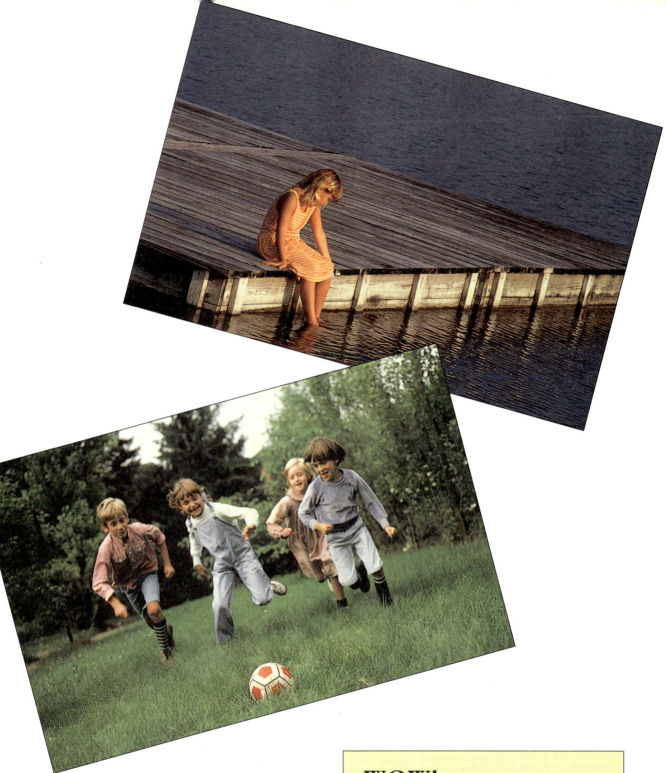

▲ Which of these children are using the most energy?

Carbohydrates

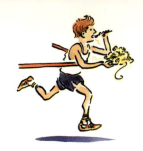

Carbohydrate foods contain a lot of starch or sugar. Too much sugar is bad for you, but starches are excellent energy foods. If you want to keep going when everyone else is getting tired, eat lots of potatoes, rice , pasta, bread and cereal. This is the kind of food that marathon runners eat before long-distance races. ▼

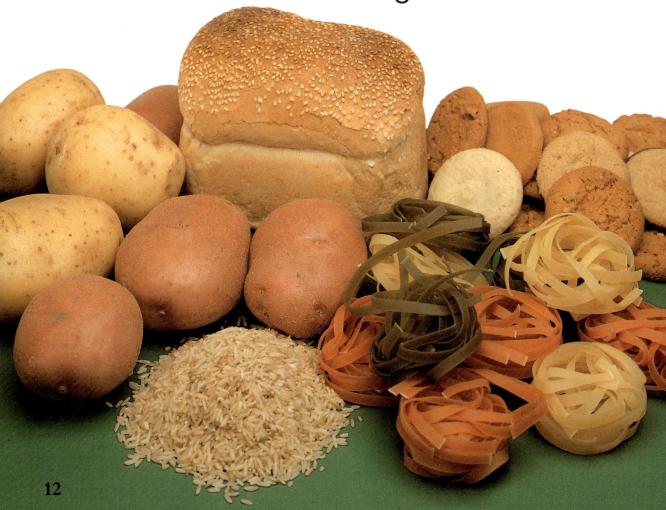

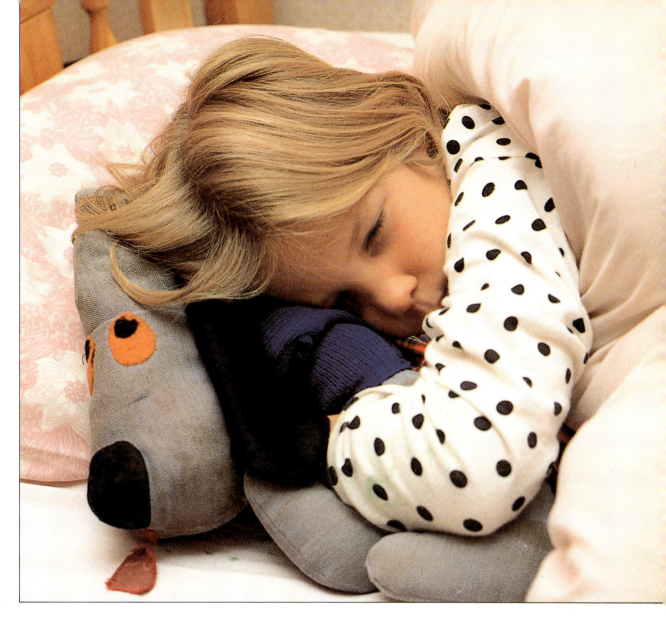

Different kinds of food give you different amounts of energy. If you do not use up all the energy you get from your food, your body stores it and so you get fat.

▲ If you do not get enough energy from your food, you become tired and ill.

Fats

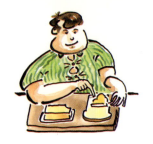

Like carbohydrates, fats give you energy to do things. You also need fats to keep you warm.

You need to eat some fat, but not too much. Try to spread butter or margarine thinly. Eat jacket potatoes instead of fatty chips.

These are the kinds of food that contain a lot of fat. ▼

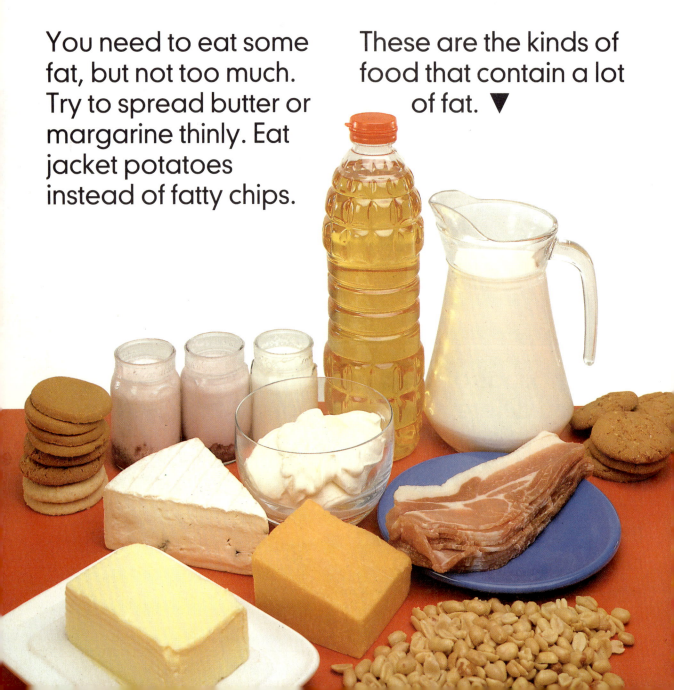

If you want to find out whether a type of food has a lot of fat in it, all you need is some brown paper. Simply rub the paper against the food, then hold the paper up to the light. If the paper goes see-through, then the food has fat in it.

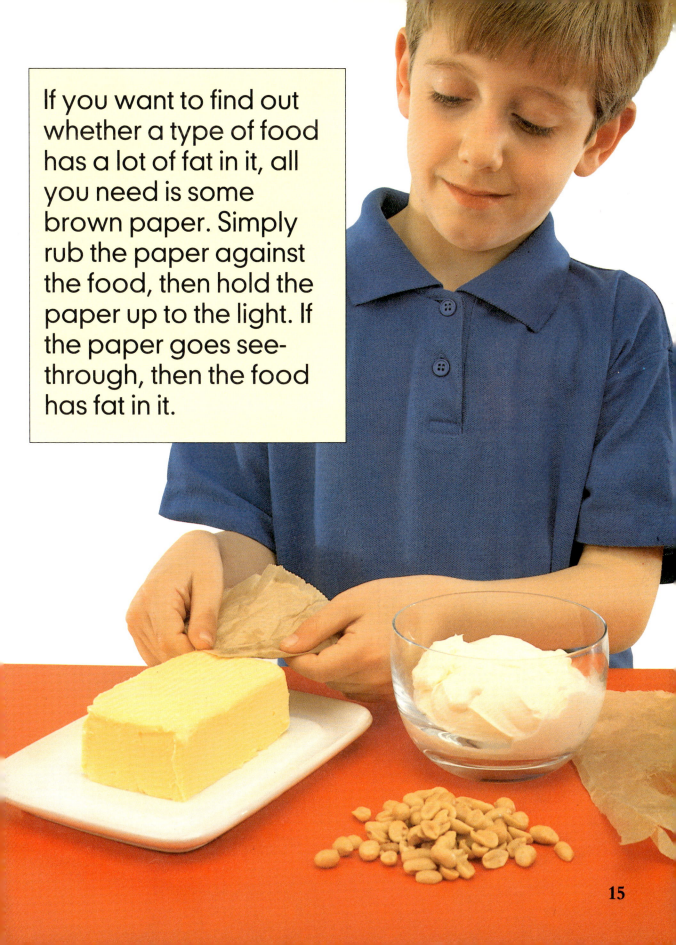

Proteins

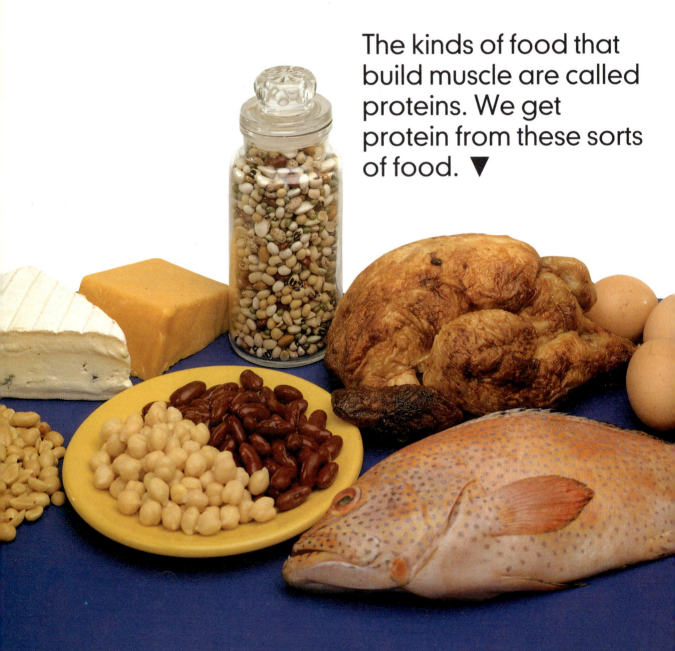

While you are still growing, you need to build more muscle. When you have finished growing, you need to replace used-up muscle.

The kinds of food that build muscle are called proteins. We get protein from these sorts of food. ▼

Where is the protein in these meals?

In the fish.

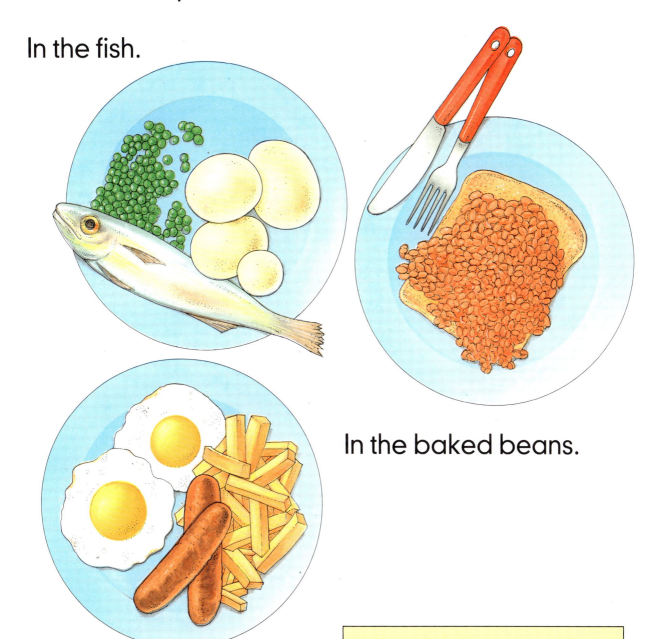

In the baked beans.

In the sausages – but they also contain a lot of fat.

WOW!
There are about 650 muscles in the human body.

Vitamins and minerals

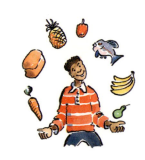

Your body needs to break up the food you eat to build body cells. To do this, you need vitamins and minerals. They are like the cement that sticks the building blocks together.

This chart shows you some of the most important vitamins and minerals. ▼

vitamin	found in...
A	cod liver oil, milk, dark green and yellow vegetables, apricots, oranges, peaches, melons
B	bread, cereal, milk, liver, unfatty meat, fish
C	citrus fruit, beans, sprouts, berries, green peppers, tomatoes
calcium	milk, cheese, yoghurt, bread, sardines, green leafy vegetables
iron	red meat, bread, eggs

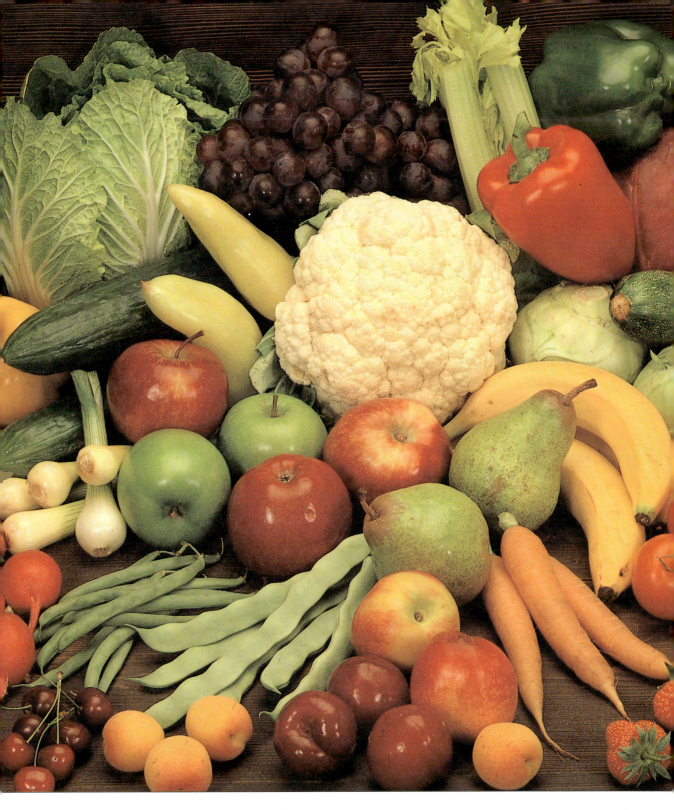

▲ Fruit and vegetables provide a lot of the vitamins and minerals which you need.

Fibre

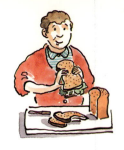

After you have swallowed your food, it is squeezed along a tube inside you. The tube keeps getting tighter and then looser.

You need to eat fibre so that the tube your food goes along can squeeze properly. Fibre comes from foods like cereal, potatoes and vegetables. ▼

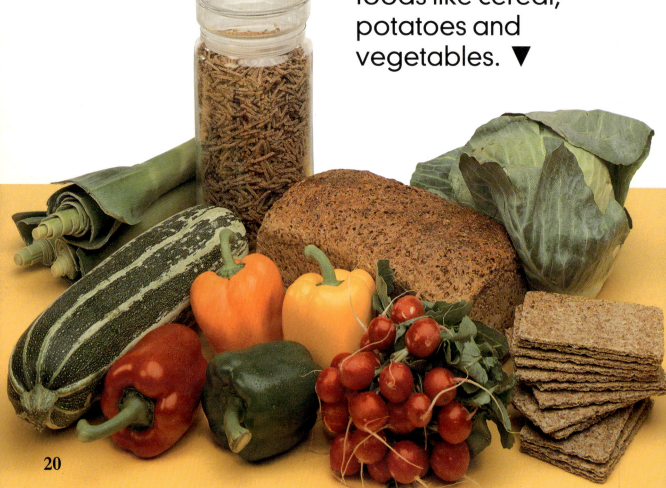

Take a long sock, a hard ball and a soft foam ball. Put the hard ball into the sock. Squeeze the sock so that the ball moves along. It's easy isn't it?
Now try the same thing with the soft ball. It's not easy is it? ▼

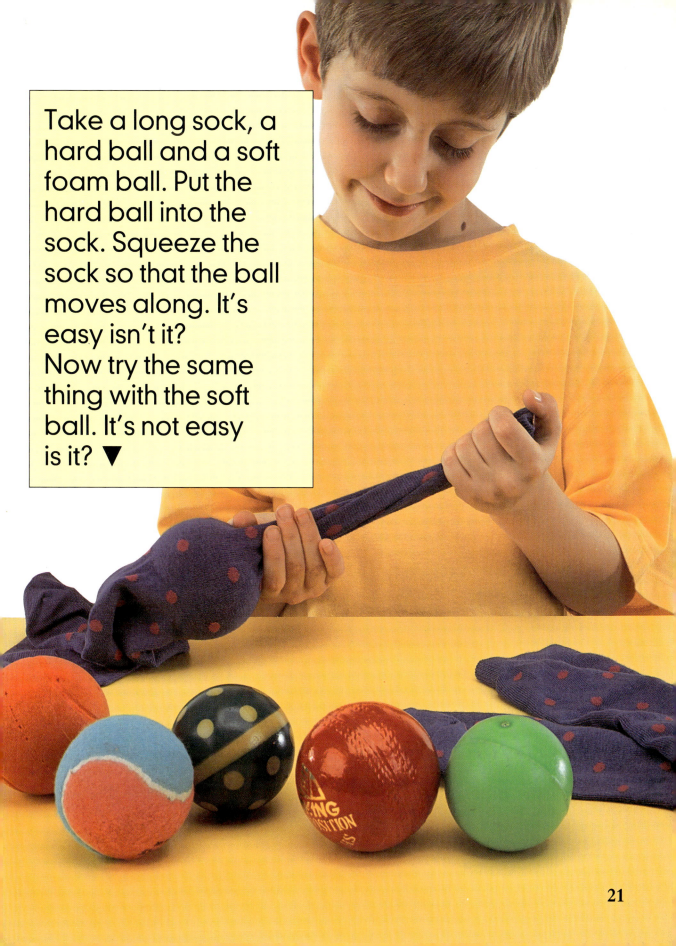

21

Around the world

All of these children are healthy. This is because they all eat balanced meals. The ideas for the meals come from all over the world.

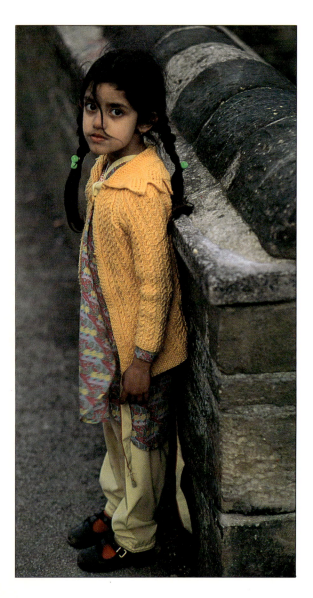

◄ This is Rucksana. Her family came from India originally, but Rucksana was born in England. Her favourite meal is *vali khichri*. This is made from rice, mung beans and spinach.

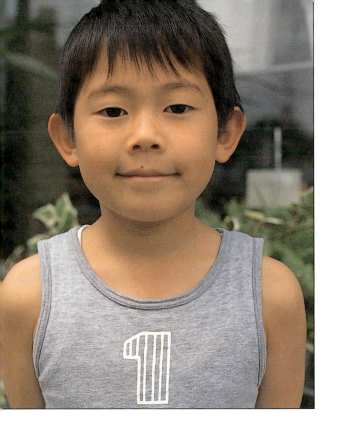

◄ This is Kenji. He is Japanese. His favourite meal is *shabu shabu* with rice. *Shabu shabu* is made from thin slices of beef dipped in vegetable soup and a sweetish sauce.

This is Maria. ► She is Italian. She likes ham pizza and salad.

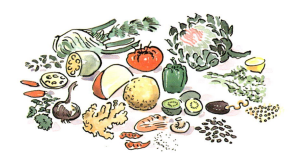

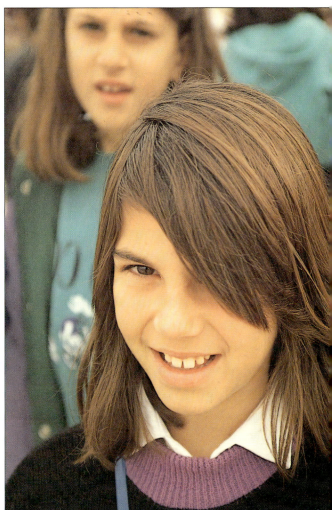

Eat safely

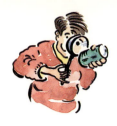

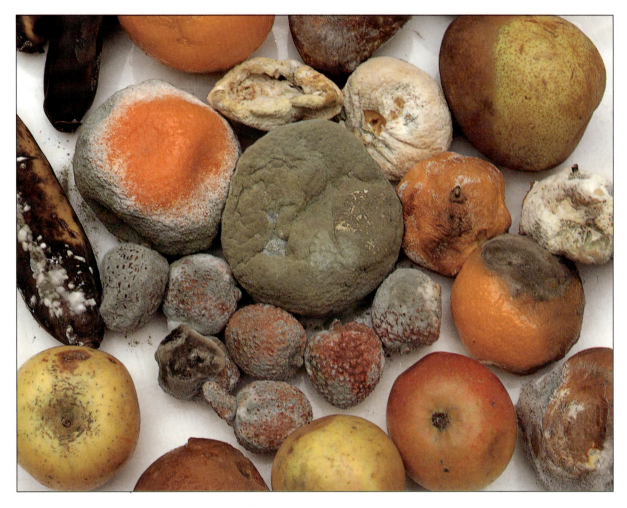

You are not the only one who likes your food. Germs do too! If they get on to your food and you eat them, they can give you food poisoning.

Sometimes you can ▲ see germs – just look at the mould on this food – but most of the time they are invisible because they are so very tiny.

Check the sell-by dates on food in your kitchen. Look at tins, packets and fresh foods like butter or milk. Which last longest?

Fresh foods usually last only a few days after opening. Unopened tins or packets last longer.

Always wash your hands before you eat, especially after going to the toilet. This will get rid of any germs. ▼

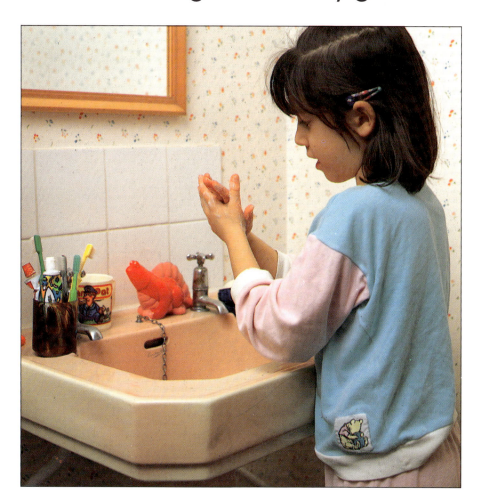

Hidden foods

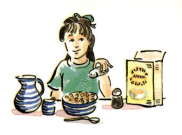

Lots of the foods in the shops have hidden ingredients in them. This makes it hard to get a properly balanced diet. You probably think of baked beans as a savoury food but in fact they contain a lot of sugar. Similarly, breakfast cereal contains salt. ▼

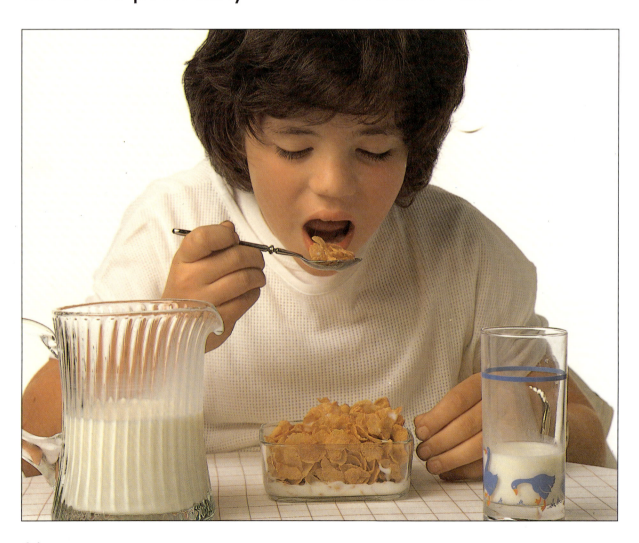

Fresh food is better for you than processed food. This is because it has no hidden ingredients.

◀ Read the contents of different types of processed food. The amount of protein, fat, starch and fibre is given in grams. What do they have most of?

WOW!
A bottle of tomato sauce can have up to twenty-seven teaspoonfuls of sugar in it.

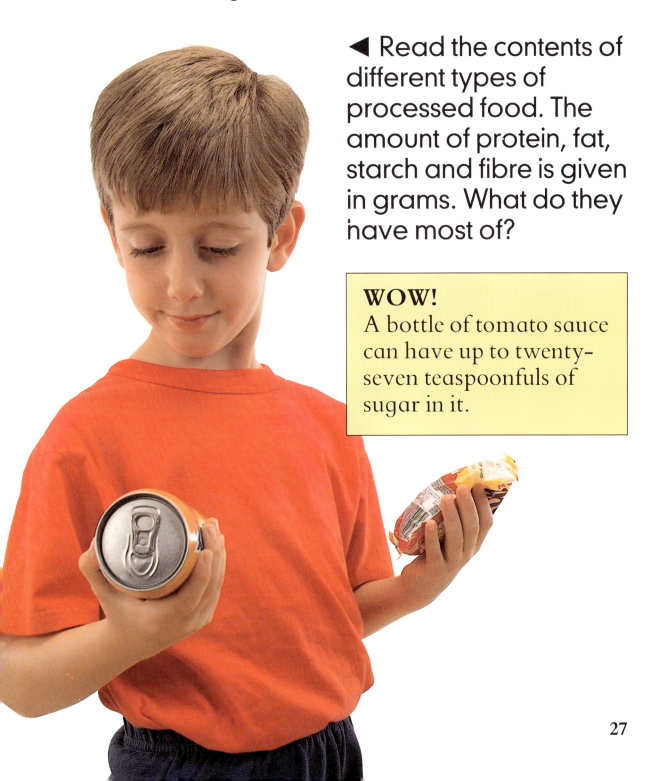

Healthy meals

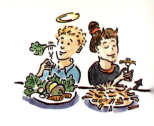

How could you make the following meals more healthy and balanced?

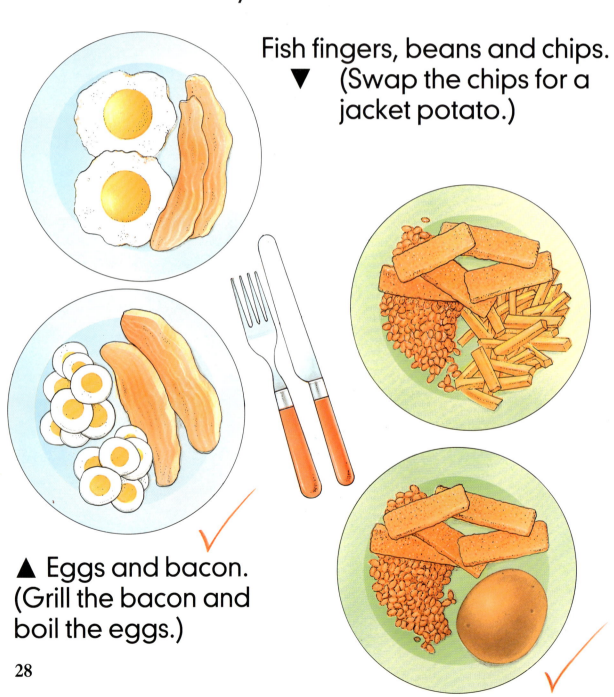

Fish fingers, beans and chips.
▼ (Swap the chips for a jacket potato.)

▲ Eggs and bacon. (Grill the bacon and boil the eggs.)

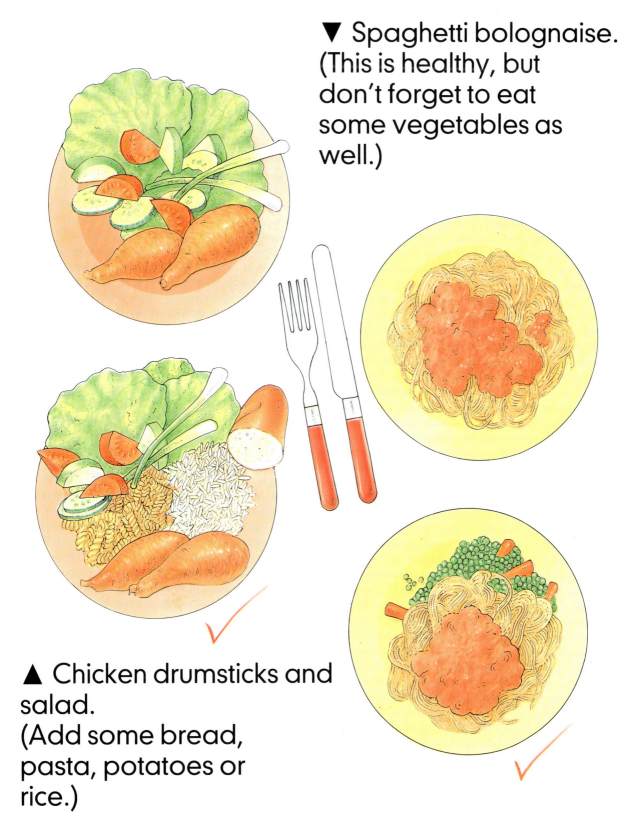

▼ Spaghetti bolognaise.
(This is healthy, but
don't forget to eat
some vegetables as
well.)

▲ Chicken drumsticks and
salad.
(Add some bread,
pasta, potatoes or
rice.)

Glossary

Calcium   A mineral which is important for healthy teeth and bones.

Carbohydrates   Foods that contain a lot of starch and sugar. They give you energy.

Cell   All living things are made up of cells. You need a microscope to be able to see them. Different parts of you are made of different types of cells.

Fats   Foods that give you energy. They can feel very greasy, such as butter.

Fibre   The part of food which is not used up by your body. Fibre helps you to push the food along inside you while it is being digested.

Iron   A mineral needed for healthy blood and muscles.

Minerals   Chemicals found in food which keep you healthy.

Protein   You need this type of food to build muscles and to repair damaged parts of your body.

Sell-by date   A date put on food wrappers. The shop must sell the food by that date.

Vitamins   Special chemicals in food which you need to stay healthy.

Books to read

There are lots of ideas in this book that you may want to explore further. Here are some books for you to read:

Food by Beverly Mathias and Ruth Thomson (Franklin Watts, 1989)
Health and Food by Dorothy Baldwin (Wayland, 1987)
Healthy Eating by Wayne Jackman (Wayland, 1990)
My Apple by Kay Davies and Wendy Oldfield (A & C Black, 1990)
What's that Taste? by Kate Perry (Franklin Watts, 1987)

Index